Title:Food For Fertility-Effective Guide To Prepare Your Body With Nutrition

BY

ROBERT DONALDSON

TABLE OF CONTENT

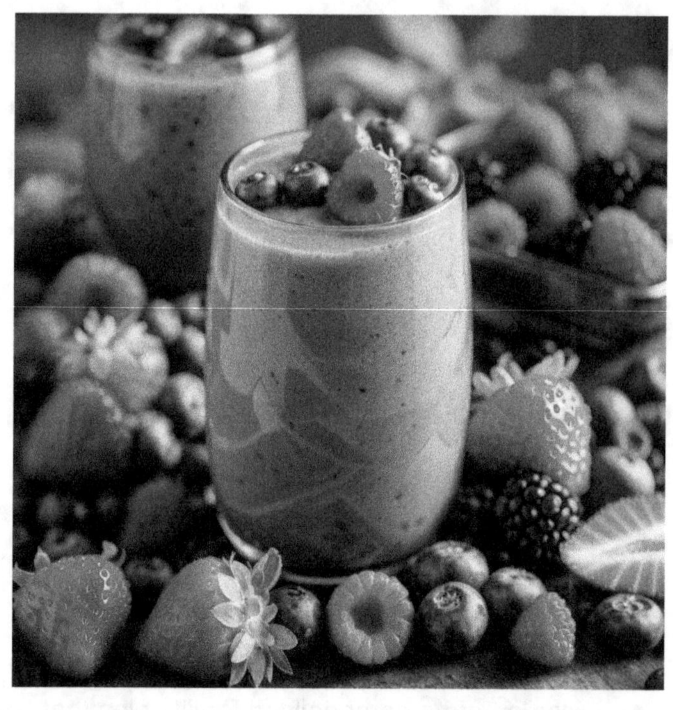

Introduction

"Welcome to Food for Fertility, your comprehensive guide to nutrition and lifestyle for optimal fertility. If you're trying to conceive,struggling with infertility, or simply looking to optimise your reproductive health, this book is for you.

When it comes to fertility, nutrition plays a critical role. The food we eat provides our bodies with the building blocks necessary for optimal reproductive health, hormone balance, and overall well-being. Yet, many of us are not getting the nutrients we need to support our fertility.

The modern diet is often high in processed foods, added sugars, and unhealthy fats, which can disrupt hormone balance, lead to inflammation, and impair fertility. Additionally, many of us are lacking in essential nutrients like omega-3 fatty acids, vitamin D, and probiotics, which are critical for fertility.

But there is hope. By focusing on whole, unprocessed foods and a balanced lifestyle, you can optimise your fertility and increase your chances of conceiving a healthy baby.Food for Fertility takes a holistic approach to fertility, exploring the powerful connection between food, nutrition, and reproductive health.

In the following pages, we'll delve into the science of fertility, exploring the key nutrients and foods that support reproductive health. We'll also discuss meal planning, snacking, and special considerations like food sensitivities and gut health. And, we'll examine the impact of stress, sleep, and exercise on fertility, providing practical tips for managing these lifestyle factors.

Whether you're just starting your fertility journey or have been trying for years, this book is designed to support and empower you every step of the way So let's get started on the path to optimal fertility and a healthy, happy pregnancy!

CHAPTER 1

Understanding Fertility and Nutrition.

Fertility is a complex process that involves the coordination of multiple bodily systems,including the reproductive,endocrine and nutritional systems.nutrition plays a critical role in supporting fertility,and well-balanced diet can help optimise reproductive health. In this section we will explore the relationship between the fertility and nutrition including the key nutrients and foods that support reproductive health.

The Science of Fertility

The capacity to conceive and bear children is known as fertility. Fertility in women is reliant on the menstrual cycle, which is controlled by hormones generated by the uterus, ovaries,and pituitary gland. The luteal phase and the follicular phase are the two phases of the menstrual cycle.
the body prepares for ovulation by growing a follicle in the ovary, which contains an egg. Ovulation occurs when the follicle ruptures, releasing the egg

into the fallopian tube. The luteal phase begins after ovulation and is characterised by the production of progesterone, which prepares the uterus for implantation of a fertilised egg.

In men, fertility is dependent on the production of healthy sperm, which are produced in the testes and mature in the epididymis. Sperm quality and quantity are critical for fertility, and factors such as diet, lifestyle, and environmental toxins can impact sperm health.

Key Nutrients for Fertility

A well-balanced diet that includes essential nutrients is critical for supporting fertility. The following nutrients are particularly important for reproductive health:

- Folic Acid: Folic acid is essential for preventing birth defects and supporting foetal development. Food sources include leafy greens, legumes, and whole grains.

- Iron: Iron is critical for healthy ovulation and sperm production. Food sources include red meat, poultry, fish, and fortified cereals.

- Omega-3 Fatty Acids: Omega-3 fatty acids support hormone production and reduce inflammation, which can impact fertility. Food sources include fatty fish, flaxseeds, and walnuts.

- Vitamin D: Vitamin D regulates hormone production and supports immune function, both of which are critical for fertility. Food sources include fatty fish, egg yolks, and fortified dairy products.

- Antioxidants: Antioxidants reduce oxidative stress and inflammation, which can impact fertility. Food sources include berries, leafy greens, and other fruits and vegetables.

- Probiotics: Probiotics support gut health, which is critical for immune function and hormone regulation, both of which impact fertility. Food sources include fermented foods such as yoghurt, kefir, and sauerkraut.

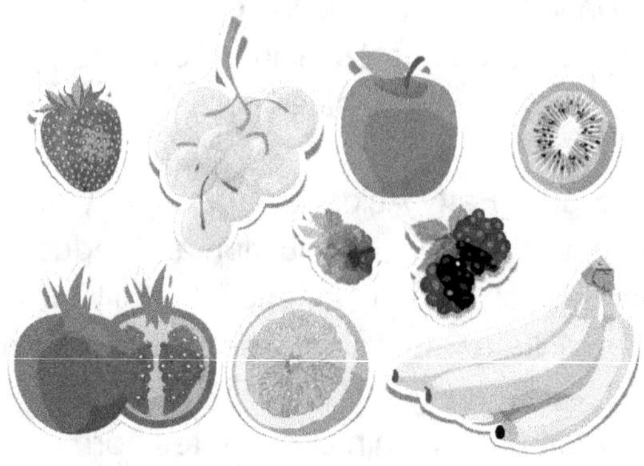

Foods that Support Fertility

In addition to essential nutrients, certain foods can support fertility due to their nutrient density and hormone-regulating properties. These foods include:

- Leafy Greens: Leafy greens such as spinach, kale, and collard greens are rich in folic acid, iron, and antioxidants.

- Berries: Berries such as blueberries, raspberries, and strawberries are rich in antioxidants and may support hormone regulation.

- Fatty Fish: Fatty fish such as salmon, sardines, and mackerel are rich in omega-3 fatty acids and vitamin D.

- Sweet Potatoes: Sweet potatoes are rich in vitamin A, which supports hormone production and immune function.

- Fermented Foods: Fermented foods such as yoghurt, kefir, and sauerkraut support gut health and immune function.

Lifestyle Factors that Impact Fertility

In addition to nutrition, lifestyle factors such as stress, sleep, and exercise can impact fertility. Chronic stress can disrupt hormone production and ovulation, while poor sleep quality can impact hormone regulation and immune function. Regular exercise can support hormone production and improve overall health, but excessive exercise can disrupt ovulation and hormone production.

The Science of Fertility

Fertility is the ability to conceive and bear children, and it is a complex process that involves the coordination of multiple bodily systems. Understanding the science of fertility is essential for individuals who are trying to conceive, as it can help them identify potential issues and take steps to optimise their reproductive health.

The Reproductive System

The reproductive system is responsible for producing sex cells (sperm and eggs) and supporting the development of a fertilised egg into a foetus. In women, the reproductive system includes the ovaries, fallopian tubes, uterus, cervix, and vagina. In men, the reproductive system includes the testes, epididymis, vas deferens, prostate gland, and urethra.

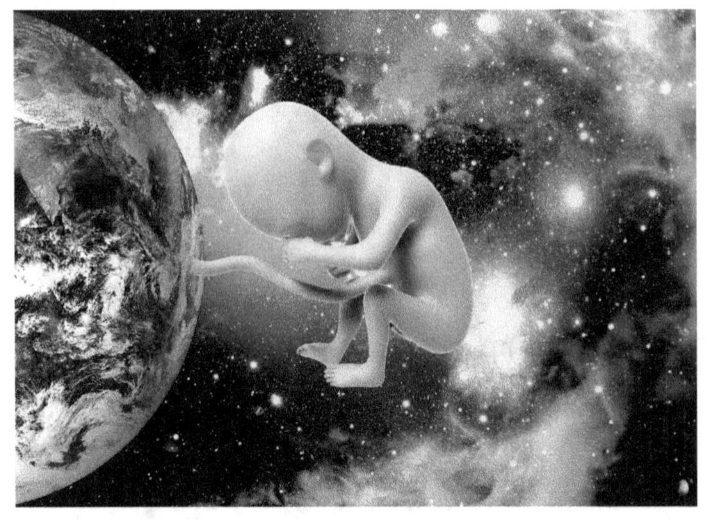

The Menstrual Cycle

The menstrual cycle is a critical aspect of fertility in women. It is a complex process that involves the coordination of hormones, ovulation, and menstruation. The menstrual cycle typically lasts around 28 days, but can vary from woman to woman. It is divided into two phases: the follicular phase and the luteal phase.

During the follicular phase, the body prepares for ovulation by growing a follicle in the ovary, which contains an egg. This phase is characterised by the production of oestrogen, which stimulates the growth of the uterine lining. Ovulation occurs when the follicle ruptures, releasing the egg into the fallopian tube.

During the luteal phase, the body prepares for implantation of a fertilised egg by producing progesterone, which maintains the uterine lining. If a pregnancy does not occur, the uterine lining sheds, resulting in menstruation.

Hormones and Fertility

Hormones play a critical role in fertility, as they regulate the menstrual cycle, ovulation, and sperm production. The key hormones involved in fertility include:

- Oestrogen: stimulates the growth of the uterine lining and prepares the body for ovulation
- Progesterone: maintains the uterine lining and prepares the body for implantation of a fertilised egg
- Follicle-stimulating hormone (FSH): stimulates the growth of follicles in the ovaries
Luteinizing hormone (LH): promotes progesterone synthesis and ovulation
- Testosterone: regulates sperm production and libido in men

Sperm Production

Sperm production is a critical aspect of fertility in men. The process of sperm production, or spermatogenesis, takes around 60-70 days and involves the following stages:

- Spermatogonia: the production of immature sperm cells
- Spermatocytes: the maturation of sperm cells
- Spermatids: the formation of sperm cells
- Spermatozoa: the mature sperm cells

Factors that Affect Fertility

Several factors can affect fertility, including:

- Age: fertility declines with age, especially after the age of 35
- Lifestyle factors: smoking, excessive alcohol consumption, and stress can impact fertility
- Medical conditions: polycystic ovary syndrome (PCOS), endometriosis, and thyroid disorders can impact fertility
- Environmental toxins: exposure to certain chemicals and pesticides can impact fertility

Nutrition and Fertility

Nutrition plays a critical role in fertility, and a well-balanced diet can help optimise reproductive health. A diet rich in essential nutrients can support hormone production, ovulation, and sperm quality, while a diet lacking in key nutrients can lead to fertility issues. In this chapter, we will explore the relationship between nutrition and fertility, including the key nutrients and foods that support reproductive health.

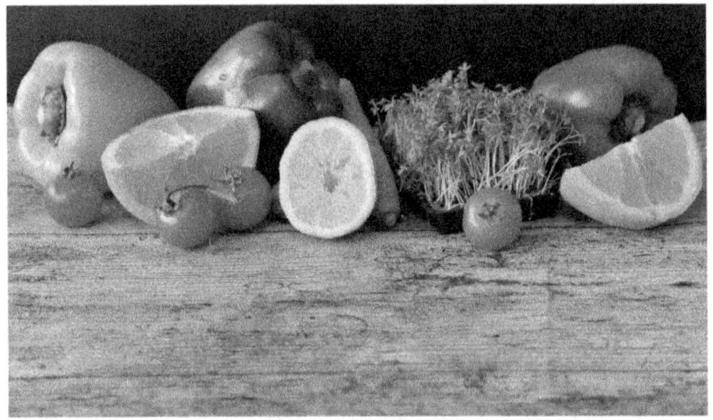

Macronutrients and Fertility

Macronutrients, including carbohydrates, protein, and fat, provide energy and support growth and development. A diet that is deficient in macronutrients can lead to fertility issues, including:

- Carbohydrates: provide energy for the body and support hormone production
- Protein: supports hormone production and ovulation
- Fat: supports hormone production and provides energy

Micronutrients, including vitamins and minerals, play a critical role in fertility. A diet that is deficient in micronutrients can lead to fertility issues, including:

- Folic acid: prevents birth defects and supports foetal development
- Iron: supports ovulation and sperm production
- Omega-3 fatty acids: supports hormone production and reduces inflammation
- Vitamin D: regulates hormone production and supports immune function
- Antioxidants: reduces oxidative stress and inflammation

Foods that Support Fertility

In addition to essential nutrients, certain foods can support fertility due to their nutrient density and hormone-regulating properties. These foods include:

- Leafy greens: rich in folic acid, iron, and antioxidants
- Berries: rich in antioxidants and may support hormone regulation
- Fatty fish: rich in omega-3 fatty acids and vitamin D
- Sweet potatoes: rich in vitamin A and fibre
- Fermented foods: supports gut health and immune function

Dietary Patterns and Fertility

Dietary patterns, including the Mediterranean diet and the fertility diet, have been shown to support fertility. These diets are characterised by:

- High intake of fruits, vegetables, and whole grains
- high consumption of omega-3 fatty acids and other healthful fats

- Low intake of processed foods and added sugars

Nutritional Deficiencies and Fertility

Nutritional deficiencies can lead to fertility issues,
including:

- Iron deficiency: can lead to anovulation and poor
sperm quality
- Vitamin D deficiency: can lead to hormonal
imbalances and poor sperm quality
- Omega-3 deficiency: can lead to hormonal
imbalances and poor sperm quality

Summary

Nutrition plays a critical role in fertility, and a well-balanced diet can help optimise reproductive health. A diet rich in essential nutrients, including macronutrients and micronutrients, can support hormone production, ovulation, and sperm quality. Foods that support fertility, including leafy greens, berries, fatty fish, sweet potatoes, and fermented foods, can also support reproductive health. Dietary patterns, including the Mediterranean diet and the fertility diet, have been shown to support fertility. Nutritional deficiencies, including iron, vitamin D, and omega-3 deficiencies, can lead to fertility issues. By understanding the relationship between nutrition and fertility, individuals can take steps to optimise their reproductive health and increase their chances of conceiving a healthy baby.

CHAPTER 2

Foods for Fertility

In this section, we will explore the real foods that can help support fertility. These foods are rich in essential nutrients, antioxidants, and other compounds that can help optimise reproductive health.

Leafy Greens and Vegetables

Leafy greens and vegetables are some of the most nutrient-dense foods on the planet. They are rich in folate, iron, and antioxidants, making them an excellent choice for supporting fertility.

- Spinach: rich in folate and iron
- Kale: rich in folate and antioxidants
- Broccoli: rich in vitamin C and antioxidants

- Carrots: rich in vitamin A and antioxidants

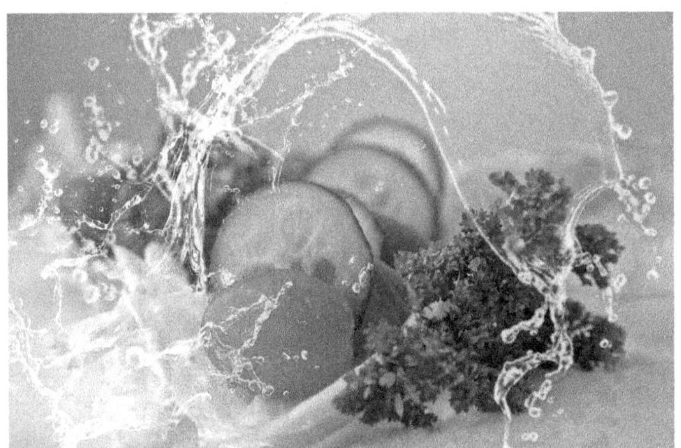

Fruits for Fertility

Fruits are a great source of antioxidants, vitamins, and minerals. They can help support hormone production, ovulation, and sperm quality.

- Berries: rich in antioxidants and may support hormone regulation
- Citrus fruits: rich in vitamin C and flavonoids
- Apples: rich in antioxidants and fibre
- Pears: rich in vitamins and minerals

Protein for Fertility

Protein is essential for hormone production, ovulation, and sperm quality. Include a source of protein in every meal to support fertility.

- Lean meats: rich in iron and zinc
- Fish: rich in omega-3 fatty acids and protein
- Eggs: rich in protein and vitamins
- Legumes: rich in protein, fibre, and minerals

Whole Grains and Legumes

Whole grains and legumes are rich in fibre, vitamins, and minerals. They can help support hormone production, ovulation, and sperm quality.

- Brown rice: rich in fibre and magnesium
- Quinoa: rich in protein and minerals
- Lentils: rich in protein and fibre
- Chickpeas: rich in protein and minerals

Healthy Fats and Oils

Healthy fats and oils are essential for hormone production, ovulation, and sperm quality. Include sources of healthy fats in your diet to support fertility.

- Avocado: rich in healthy fats and antioxidants
- Nuts and seeds: rich in healthy fats and antioxidants
- Olive oil: rich in healthy fats and antioxidants
- Fatty fish: rich in omega-3 fatty

Summary

foods can play a critical role in supporting fertility. By incorporating leafy greens, fruits, protein, whole grains, and healthy fats into your diet, you can help optimise reproductive health and increase your chances of conceiving a healthy baby. Remember to always choose whole, unprocessed foods whenever possible, and vary your diet to ensure you are getting a broad range of essential nutrients.

CHAPTER 3

Meal Planning and Snacking

Meal planning and snacking are crucial components of a fertility-friendly diet. By planning your meals and snacks in advance, you can ensure that you are getting the nutrients you need to support reproductive health. In this section, we will explore the importance of meal planning and snacking, and provide tips and ideas for incorporating these habits into your daily routine.

Breakfast for Fertility

Breakfast is the most important meal of the day, and it's especially crucial when it comes to fertility. A fertility-friendly breakfast should include a balance of protein, healthy fats, and complex carbohydrates.

- Overnight oats with fruit and nuts
- whole wheat bread and spinach in scrambled eggs
- Avocado toast with poached eggs and cherry tomatoes

Lunch and Dinner Ideas

Lunch and dinner should include a balance of protein, healthy fats, and complex carbohydrates, as well as a variety of fruits and vegetables.

- Grilled chicken salad with mixed greens, berries, and walnuts
- Bowl of quinoa, black beans, roasted veggies, and avocado
- Baked salmon with sweet potato and green beans

Snacking for Fertility

Snacking can help keep your energy levels up and prevent nutrient deficiencies. Choose snacks that are rich in protein, healthy fats, and complex carbohydrates.

- Fresh fruit and nuts
- Energy balls consisting of almonds, dried fruit, and oats
- Hard-boiled eggs and veggies

Meal Planning Tips

You may save money, stress, and time by organising your meals. The following advice can help you make meal planning a regular part of your schedule: - Arrange your weekly menu in advance.
- Make a grocery list and stick to it
- Prep meals in advance, such as cooking a big batch of rice or quinoa
- Use a slow cooker or instant pot to make meal prep easy

Snack Planning Tips

Snack planning can help you make healthy choices and avoid nutrient deficiencies. Here are some tips for incorporating snack planning into your routine:

- Plan your snacks for the day ahead of time
- Keep healthy snacks on hand, such as nuts and dried fruit
- Prep snacks in advance, such as cutting up veggies and fruit
- Use a snack container or bag to keep snacks organised and portable

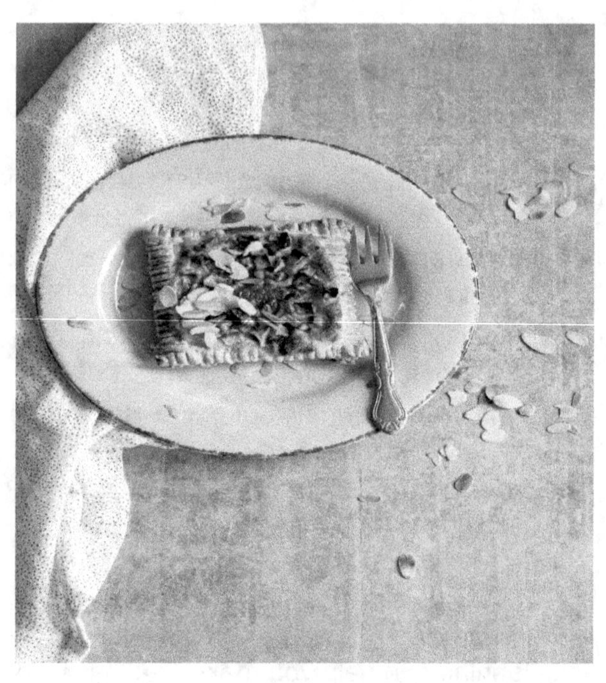

Summary

Meal planning and snacking are crucial components of a fertility-friendly diet. By planning your meals and snacks in advance, you can ensure that you are getting the nutrients you need to support reproductive health. Remember to choose whole, unprocessed foods whenever possible, and vary your diet to ensure you are getting a broad range of essential nutrients. With a little planning and prep, you can support your fertility and overall health.

CHAPTER 4

Special Considerations

While a fertility-friendly diet is essential for optimal reproductive health, there are certain special considerations that need to be taken into account. In this section, we will explore these special considerations and provide guidance on how to navigate them.

Food Sensitivities and Allergies

Food sensitivities and allergies can have a significant impact on fertility. Common culprits include gluten, dairy, and soy.

- Identify and avoid trigger foods
- Incorporate gut-healing foods like bone broth and probiotics
- Consider working with a healthcare provider or registered dietitian to develop a personalised plan

Vegetarian and Vegan Diets

Vegetarian and vegan diets can be fertility-friendly, but require careful planning to ensure adequate nutrient intake.

- Incorporate plant-based sources of protein like legumes and nuts
- Choose whole grains and a variety of colourful vegetables
- Think about taking iron and vitamin B12 supplements.

Gut Health and Fertility

Gut health is critical for fertility, as the gut microbiome plays a key role in hormone regulation and nutrient absorption.

- Take vitamin B12 and iron supplements into consideration.
- Consider taking a probiotic supplement
- Avoid foods that can disrupt the gut microbiome, like added sugars and processed foods

Stress and Fertility

Stress can have a significant impact on fertility, as it can disrupt hormone balance and ovulation.

- Include methods for lowering stress, such as deep breathing and meditation.
- Prioritise self-care and relaxation
- Consider working with a healthcare provider or therapist to develop a stress management plan

Supplements and Fertility

Supplements can be a helpful addition to a fertility-friendly diet, but it's essential to choose high-quality options and consult with a healthcare provider before starting any new supplements.

- Omega-3 fatty acids
- Vitamin D
- Probiotics
- Prenatal vitamins

Summary

Special considerations like food sensitivities, vegetarian and vegan diets, gut health, stress, and supplements can have a significant impact on fertility. By understanding and addressing these factors, individuals can optimise their reproductive health and increase their chances of conceiving a healthy baby. Remember to always consult with a healthcare provider or registered dietitian for personalised guidance and support.

CHAPTER 5

Lifestyle and Stress Management

Lifestyle and stress management are critical components of a fertility-friendly plan. In addition to a balanced diet, incorporating healthy lifestyle habits and stress-reducing techniques can help optimise reproductive health. In this section, we will explore the importance of lifestyle and stress management for fertility and provide tips and ideas for incorporating these habits into daily life.

Exercise and Fertility

Regular exercise can help improve fertility by reducing stress, promoting weight management, and improving overall health.

- Aim for 30 minutes of moderate-intensity exercise per day
- Incorporate strength training and high-intensity interval training (HIIT)
- Consider working with a personal trainer or fitness coach to develop a personalised exercise plan

Sleep and Fertility

Adequate sleep is essential for fertility, as it helps regulate hormones and support overall health.

- Sleep for 7-8 hours every night is the goal.
- Establish a relaxing bedtime routine
- Create a sleep-conducive environment, such as keeping the bedroom cool and dark

Chapter 20: Stress Management and Fertility

Stress can have a significant impact on fertility, as it can disrupt hormone balance and ovulation.

- Include methods for lowering stress, such as deep breathing and meditation.
- Prioritise self-care and relaxation
- Consider working with a healthcare provider or therapist to develop a stress management plan

Chapter 21: Environmental Toxins and Fertility

Environmental toxins can have a negative impact on fertility, as they can disrupt hormone balance and overall health.

- Avoid exposure to chemicals like BPA and
phthalates
- Make use of non-toxic personal care and
household cleaning products.
- Consider working with a healthcare provider or
environmental health specialist to develop a plan for
reducing exposure to environmental toxins

Social Support and Fertility

Social support can have a positive impact on
fertility, as it can help reduce stress and promote
overall well-being.

- Create a network of friends, family, and medical
professionals for support.
- Consider joining a fertility support group
- Prioritise self-care and relaxation

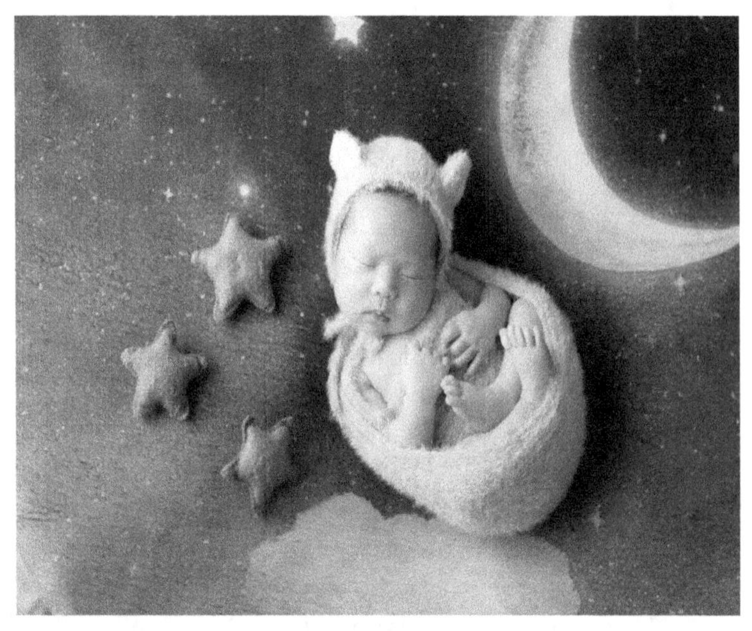

Summary

Lifestyle and stress management are critical components of a fertility-friendly plan. By incorporating healthy lifestyle habits and stress-reducing techniques, individuals can optimise their reproductive health and increase their chances of conceiving a healthy baby. Remember to always consult with a healthcare provider or registered dietitian for personalised guidance and support.

Chapter 6

Putting it All Together

Congratulations on reaching the final part of our comprehensive guide to fertility! By now, you have a solid understanding of the importance of nutrition, lifestyle, and stress management for optimal reproductive health. In this final section, we will put it all together and provide a step-by-step guide on how to implement a fertility-friendly plan into your daily life.

Step 1: Set Your Fertility Goals

- Define your fertility goals and priorities
- Identify any challenges or obstacles you may face
- Create a timeline for achieving your goals

Step 2: Assess Your Current Lifestyle

- Evaluate your current diet and nutrition habits
- Assess your physical activity level and exercise routine

- Identify sources of stress and anxiety in your life

Step 3: Create a Personalized Fertility Plan

- Based on your goals and assessment, create a
personalised plan that includes:
- Nutrition and meal planning
- Lifestyle changes and stress management
techniques
- Supplements and vitamins (if necessary)
- Regular exercise and physical activity
- Making an appointment for routine check-ins
with your physician

Step 4: Implement Your Plan

- Start implementing your plan gradually, making
small changes at a time
- Be consistent and patient, as it may take time to
see results
- Don't be too hard on yourself if you encounter
setbacks - simply get back on track

Step 5: Monitor Your Progress

- Monitor your progress and make any necessary adjustments to your plan.
- Celebrate your successes and don't be discouraged by setbacks
- Remember that fertility is a journey, and it may take time to achieve your goals

Additional Tips:

- Stay informed and educated about fertility and reproductive health
- Seek support from loved ones, support groups, or online resources
- Remember to prioritise self-care and stress management

Congratulations on completing our comprehensive guide to fertility! By following these steps and putting it all together, you can create a personalised fertility plan that works for you. Remember to stay patient, consistent, and informed, and don't hesitate to seek support when needed. Good luck on your fertility journey!

Optimising fertility requires a comprehensive approach that incorporates a balanced diet, healthy lifestyle habits, and effective stress management techniques.
food for fertility provides the essential nutrients, antioxidants, and hormonal support necessary for optimal reproductive health. By focusing on whole, unprocessed foods and avoiding harmful substances, individuals can improve their chances of conceiving and maintaining a healthy pregnancy.

Key takeaways:

- Eat a variety of whole, unprocessed foods including leafy greens, berries, fatty fish, and whole grains
- Avoid harmful substances like added sugars, processed foods, and excessive caffeine and alcohol
- Stay hydrated and limit exposure to environmental toxins
- Include methods for lowering stress, such as deep breathing and meditation.
- Prioritise sleep and aim for 7-8 hours per night
- Think about taking probiotics, vitamin D, and omega-3 fatty acids as supplements.

By incorporating these principles into daily life, individuals can support their fertility and overall health, increasing their chances of conceiving and maintaining a healthy pregnancy. Remember, fertility is a journey, and patience, consistency, and self-care are essential for success.

www.ingramcontent.com/pod-product-compliance
Lightning Source LLC
Chambersburg PA
CBHW051712250726
48653CB00007B/2982